GASTRIC SLEEVE DIET PLAN GUIDE BOOK

Nourishing Your New Stomach: An Complete Handbook on the Gastric Sleeve Diet

REX LEWIS

Introduction

The Gastric Sleeve Diet Is An Essential Part Of The Care Before And After Gastric Sleeve Surgery, Also Called Sleeve Gastrectomy. This Surgical Procedure Entails Excising A Substantial Portion Of The Stomach, Resulting In A Smaller, Banana-Shaped Stomach Pouch. The Decrease In Stomach Capacity Restricts Food Intake, Resulting In Weight Reduction.

The Gastric Sleeve Diet Serves Many Functions Within The Comprehensive Treatment Regimen For Persons Following This Surgery. Prior To The Surgery, Patients Usually Need To Adhere To A Specialized Diet To Reduce The Size Of The Liver, Since An

Enlarged Liver Can Complicate The Surgical Process. The Pre-Operative Diet Often Includes A Low-Calorie, High-Protein Strategy To Promote Weight Loss And Minimize The Chances Of Problems During The Surgical Procedure.

Following Gastric Sleeve Surgery, Patients Choose A Post-Operative Diet Designed To Facilitate Healing, Minimize Problems, And Encourage Steady Weight Reduction. During The Early Post-Operative Period, Patients Usually Follow A Liquid Or Pureed Diet To Facilitate Stomach Healing. Patients Gradually Transition From Soft To Solid Foods, Gradually

Reintroducing A Range Of Foods While Maintaining Portion Control.

Essential Elements Of The Gastric Sleeve Diet Often Consist Of:

• Protein Is Crucial For The Recovery Process And Preserving Muscular Mass. The Diet Focuses On Lean Protein Sources Such Poultry, Fish, Eggs, And Dairy.

• Low Carbohydrate Intake Involves Focusing On Consuming Complex Carbs And Avoiding Simple Sweets To Regulate Blood Sugar Levels And Aid In Weight Loss, Rather Than Completely Eliminating Carbohydrates.

- Staying Well-Hydrated Is Essential For Good Health, And It Is Recommended That Persons Drink A Certain Amount Of Water Daily.

- Patients With Reduced Stomach Size And Altered Nutrient Absorption May Need To Take Vitamin And Mineral Supplements To Avoid Deficits.

- Portion Control Is Crucial In The Diet After Surgery Due To The Reduced Capacity Of The Stomach, Helping To Prevent Overeating And Facilitate Weight Loss.

- The Diet Progresses Gradually From Liquids to Pureed Foods, Soft Foods, And Solid Foods, Enabling The

Stomach To Adjust To Various Textures And Consistencies.

It Is Essential For Patients Having Gastric Sleeve Surgery To Strictly Stick To Their Healthcare Provider's Diet Plan Suggestions, As Following Dietary Advice Is Critical For Attaining Successful Weight Loss And Sustaining Long-Term Health. Furthermore, Continuous Dietary Advice And Assistance Are Frequently Offered To Assist Patients In Making Lasting Lifestyle Modifications.

CHAPTER ONE
Comprehending the Gastric Sleeve Surgery

The Gastric Sleeve Operation, Also Called Sleeve Gastrectomy, Is A Surgical Weight-Loss Method Where A Significant Piece Of The Stomach Is Removed To Form A Smaller, Sleeve-Shaped Stomach. This Operation Aims To Facilitate Substantial Weight Loss By Limiting The Stomach's Food Capacity And Modifying Hormonal Cues Linked To Appetite And Fullness.

Here Is A Detailed Explanation Of The Gastric Sleeve Procedure:

Preoperative Preparation:

• **Medical Assessment:** Prior To The Procedure, Individuals Receive A Comprehensive Medical Evaluation, Which Includes Assessments Of General Health, Obesity-Related Conditions, And Dietary Status.

• Patients Frequently Need To Adhere To A Prescribed Diet And Exercise Regimen Before Undergoing Surgery. Prior To Surgery, Weight Loss May Be Necessary To Decrease Liver Size And Aid In The Surgical Process.

Surgery:

• **Anesthesia:** The Patient Is Administered General Anesthesia To

Induce Unconsciousness And Eliminate Pain Sensation During The Surgical Procedure.

• **Incisions:** Usually, The Procedure Is Carried Out Utilizing Minimally Invasive Laparoscopic Procedures. Small Cuts Are Created In The Abdomen To Introduce A Laparoscope And Specialized Surgical Tools.

• During A Stomach Resection, The Surgeon Eliminates Around 75-80% Of The Stomach Along The Larger Curvature, Resulting In A Narrow, Tubular Structure That Resembles A Banana Or Sleeve. The Remaining Portion Of The Stomach Is Closed Off Using Surgical Staples.

• To Prevent Leaks Or Difficulties, The Suture Line Is Frequently Strengthened With Extra Sutures Or Staples.

• The Excised Section Of The Stomach Is Removed From The Abdominal Cavity.

• Conclusion: Once Confirming The Absence Of Bleeding Or Problems, The Incisions Are Sealed Using Stitches Or Staples.

Recovery after Surgery:

• **Hospital Stay:** Patients Usually Stay One To Two Days In The Hospital For Initial Recovery And Monitoring.

- The Post-Operative Diet Advances Gradually From Clear Liquids To Pureed Foods, Soft Foods, And Finally Solid Foods Over A Period Of Weeks. This Sequence Enables The Stomach To Recover And Adjust To The Smaller Size.

- Regular Follow-Up Consultations With The Surgical Team Are Scheduled For Monitoring Progress, Addressing Issues, And Providing Continuous Support.

Long-Term Alterations:

- The Gastric Sleeve Treatment Facilitates Weight Loss By Limiting Food Intake, Resulting In Decreased Calorie Consumption.

• The Operation Modifies Hormonal Signals That Regulate Hunger And Fullness, Leading To Reduced Appetite And Better Management Of Eating Behaviors.

• To Achieve Lasting Success, It Is Essential To Acquire And Sustain Healthy Lifestyle Habits Such As Consistent Physical Activity, A Well-Rounded Diet, And Continuous Medical Monitoring.

It Is Crucial To Understand That The Gastric Sleeve Surgery Can Be Quite Beneficial For Weight Loss, But It Is A Major Decision That Should Be Discussed With Healthcare Specialists. The Treatment Is Permanent, And

Anyone Contemplating It Should Be Ready For Enduring Alterations In Diet And Lifestyle. Post-Operative Support, Such As Nutritional Counseling And Psychiatric Aid, Is Frequently A Crucial Component Of The Comprehensive Treatment Strategy.

Significance of a Correct Diet after Surgery

Following Gastric Sleeve Surgery Or Any Weight-Loss Surgery, Maintaining A Good Diet Is Crucial. The Diet After Surgery Is Essential For A Successful Recovery, Reducing Problems, And Promoting Long-Term Weight Loss And General Health Advantages. Here Are Key Reasons Emphasizing The

Significance Of A Good Diet After Surgery:

• **Facilitates Healing:** Adhering To A Recommended Diet Aids In The Recovery Post Gastric Sleeve Surgery. The Stomach Requires Time To Adapt To Its Altered Size And Shape. Following A Well-Thought-Out Diet Helps Avoid Putting Stress On The Surgical Area, Thereby Lowering The Chances Of Issues Like Leaks Or Infections.

• The Smaller Stomach Size Can Hinder The Body's Absorption Of Specific Nutrients, Perhaps Leading To Nutritional Deficiencies. An Adequately Balanced Diet Following

Surgery, Typically Enhanced With Vitamins And Minerals, Aids In Averting Nutritional Deficits, Guaranteeing The Body Obtains Vital Elements For Peak Health.

• Gastric Sleeve Surgery Aims To Accomplish Substantial Weight Loss. Following A Suitable Post-Operative Diet That Begins With Liquids And Advances To Solid Foods Gradually Helps Individuals Control Their Caloric Intake, Avoiding Overeating And Promoting Steady, Consistent Weight Loss.

• **Adjusts To Stomach Capacity:** The Decreased Size Of The Stomach Restricts Individuals From Consuming

Huge Amounts Of Food. Adhering To A Suitable Diet After Surgery Instructs Individuals On Managing Portion Sizes And Assists Them In Adjusting To Their Reduced Stomach Capacity, Reducing Discomfort And Enhancing Satisfaction With Smaller Meals.

• **Reduces Discomfort And Complications**: A Properly Planned Diet Decreases Discomfort, Nausea, And Other Digestive Problems That May Occur If Unsuitable Foods Are Eaten Shortly After Surgery. It Also Aids In Preventing Complications Including Dumping Syndrome, A Condition Characterized By Rapid Movement Of Food From The Stomach To The Small Intestine.

- **Facilitates Enduring Lifestyle Modifications:** Postoperative Dietary Recommendations Are Not Transient; They Establish The Groundwork For Sustained Lifestyle Alterations. Adopting Healthy Eating Habits, Selecting Nutritious Foods, And Following A Balanced Diet Are Key Factors For Achieving Long-Term Weight Loss And Improving Overall Health.

- Gastric Sleeve Surgery Facilitates Behavior Modification By Altering Both The Physical Processes Of Digestion And Hormonal Signals Associated With Hunger And Satiety. Adhering To A Suitable Diet Assists Patients In Identifying And Reacting

To These Signals, Which Aids In Behavior Adjustment And Promotes Healthy Eating Habits.

• **Reduces The Risk Of Complications:** Adequate Nutrition After Surgery Decreases The Likelihood Of Complications Such Starvation, Dehydration, And Gastrointestinal Problems. Consistent Monitoring Of Nutrient Levels And Following Dietary Guidelines Help Improve Recuperation And Enhance Overall Health Results.

• A Balanced Diet Boosts Energy Levels and Overall Well-Being By Providing Essential Nutrients For Daily Tasks, Therefore Minimizing

Weariness. Sufficient Nourishment Aids in the Body's Operations, Such As Immune System Activity And Tissue Healing.

• Adhering To the Recommended Post-Operative Diet Promotes Efficient Collaboration With Healthcare Providers. Regular Follow-Up Appointments Allow For Monitoring Progress, Addressing Issues, And Making Any Adjustments To The Eating Plan.

Essentially, A Well-Balanced Diet Following Gastric Sleeve Surgery Is Crucial For A Good Recovery, Consistent Weight Loss, And General Well-Being. Patients Must Strictly

Follow The Dietary Advice Given By Their Healthcare Team And Seek Continuous Support To Make A Seamless Transition To A Healthier Lifestyle.

Getting Ready For the Gastric Sleeve Procedure

Preparing For The Gastric Sleeve Procedure Requires Meticulous Preparation, Knowledge, And Lifestyle Changes. Below Are Essential Steps To Assist Folks In Preparing For Gastric Sleeve Surgery:

1. Medical Assessment:

• Schedule Consultations with Healthcare Professionals, Such As A Bariatric Surgeon, Dietitian, And Other

Necessary Specialists. Share Your Medical Background, Objectives For Weight Reduction, And Any Worries You May Have.

• **Health Assessments:** Complete Thorough Health Assessments To Establish Your Suitability For Gastric Sleeve Surgery. Evaluations May Consist Of Physical Exams, Blood Tests, And Imaging Scans.

2. Education and Counseling:

• Participate In Bariatric Seminars Or Support Groups: Healthcare Professionals Often Arrange Informative Seminars Or Support Groups For Those Contemplating Weight-Loss Surgery. Participate In

These Sessions To Gain Knowledge About The Process, Anticipated Results, And Adjustments To Lifestyle.

- **Nutritional Counseling:** Consult With A Trained Dietitian Or Nutritionist To Learn About Dietary Needs Before And After Surgery. Explore Portion Control, Nutrient-Dense Meals, And The Significance Of Establishing Sustainable Nutritional Practices.

- **Behavioral Counseling:** Utilize Behavioral Counseling To Target Emotional And Psychological Aspects Associated With Eating Patterns. Acquire Coping Mechanisms And Cultivate A Supportive Mindset For The Journey.

3. Changes in Lifestyle:

- **Diet and Exercise:** Begin Making Moderate Modifications To Your Diet And Exercise Program Before Surgery. Adopt A Balanced, Nutrient-Rich Diet And Engage In Regular Physical Activity To Promote General Health And Ease Pre-Operative Weight Loss.

- **Smoking Cessation And Alcohol Moderation:** If Applicable, Consider Quitting Smoking And Regulating Alcohol Use. Both Smoking And Excessive Alcohol Intake Might Raise The Risk Of Problems And May Affect The Outcome Of The Procedure.

4. Pre-Operative Diet:

• **Follow Pre-Operative Dietary Advice:** Your Healthcare Provider Will Likely Advise Particular Dietary Advice To Follow Before Surgery. This May Include A Low-Calorie, High-Protein Diet To Shrink The Liver And Lower The Chance Of Problems During The Surgery.

• **Hydration:** Stay Well-Hydrated In The Weeks Leading Up To Surgery. Proper Hydration Is Vital For Overall Health And Can Enhance The Body's Preparation For The Next Surgery.

5. Emotional and Social Support:

- **Build A Support System:** Inform Friends And Family About Your Intention To Undergo Gastric Sleeve Surgery. Build A Support Structure To Provide Emotional Support, Encouragement, And Aid During The Healing Time.

- **Address Emotional Eating:** If Emotional Eating Is A Concern, Concentrate On Creating Alternative Coping Processes And Tactics With The Aid Of Mental Health Professionals.

6. Practical Preparations:

• **Plan For Healing**: Arrange For A Supportive Atmosphere Throughout The Initial Healing Period. Ensure You Have Assistance With Everyday Tasks, Transportation To Medical Visits, And Any Necessary Accommodations At Home.

• **Understand Insurance Coverage:** Confirm The Details Of Your Insurance Coverage For The Procedure And Associated Charges. Be Aware Of Any Pre-Authorization Requirements And Financial Responsibilities.

7. Post-Operative Planning:

• **Meal Preparation:** Plan and Prepare For the Post-Operative Diet. Stock Up On Recommended Foods, And Consider Cooking Meals In Advance For The Initial Recovery Phase.

• **Follow-Up Appointments:** Schedule and Plan For Post-Operative Follow-Up Appointments With Your Healthcare Team. Regular Monitoring And Assistance Are Necessary For Long-Term Success.

By Taking A Complete And Proactive Approach To Preparation, Individuals Can Build The Basis For A Successful Gastric Sleeve Journey. Open Communication With Healthcare

Providers, Commitment To Lifestyle Modifications, And A Strong Support Network Contribute To A Happy And Effective Experience.

CHAPTER TWO
Pre-Surgery Nutrition Guidelines

Pre-Surgical Nutrition Is A Vital Component Of The Preparation For Gastric Sleeve Surgery. Following Specific Criteria Helps Optimize Health, Limit Surgical Risks, And Prepare The Body For The Changes Involved With The Treatment. **Here Are Some Eating Suggestions Commonly Recommended Before Gastric Sleeve Surgery:**

1. High-Protein Diet:

• **Importance:** Protein Is Necessary For Tissue Repair, Immunological Function, And Muscle Preservation. A High-Protein Diet Helps Prevent

Muscle Loss And Supports Healing After Surgery.

- **Sources:** Include Lean Protein Sources Such As Poultry, Fish, Lean Meats, Eggs, Dairy, Tofu, Lentils, And Protein Supplements As Prescribed By Your Healthcare Team.

2. Low-Calorie Diet:

- **Purpose:** Reducing Calorie Consumption Helps Induce Weight Loss Before Surgery, Which Can Shrink The Size Of The Liver And Reduce The Risk Of Problems During The Treatment.

- **Focus On Nutrient Density:** While Restricting Calories, Prioritize

Nutrient-Dense Foods To Ensure That Important Vitamins And Minerals Are Still Obtained.

3. Hydration:

- **Maintain Adequate Hydration:** Drink Plenty Of Water Throughout The Day To Keep Well-Hydrated. Proper Hydration Is Vital For Overall Health And Can Help Prepare The Body For Surgery.

- **Limit Beverages With Calories:** Minimize The Intake Of Sugary Beverages, Sodas, And High-Calorie Drinks.

4. Vitamin and Mineral Supplements:

• **Follow Healthcare Practitioner Recommendations:** Depending On Individual Needs, Your Healthcare Practitioner May Recommend Specific Vitamin And Mineral Supplements To Address Potential Deficiencies And Maximize Nutritional Status.

5. Limit Sugars And Simple Carbohydrates:

• **Purpose:** Restricting Sugars And Simple Carbohydrates Helps Manage Blood Sugar Levels And Improves Weight Loss.

- **Choose Complex Carbohydrates:** Opt For Whole Grains, Fruits, And Vegetables Over Processed Carbohydrates.

6. Avoid High-Fat Foods:

- **Purpose:** Limiting High-Fat Foods Can Help Lower The Risk Of Problems During Surgery And Improve Overall Health.

- **Choose Healthy Fats:** If Including Fats, Focus On Healthy Sources Such As Avocados, Nuts, Seeds, And Olive Oil In Moderation.

7. Caffeine and Alcohol:

- **Limit Intake:** Reduce Or Eliminate Caffeine And Alcohol Intake, As They

Can Affect Hydration And May Have An Impact On The Liver.

8. Meal Timing:

• **Regular Meals and Snacks:** Aim For Regular, Balanced Meals And Snacks To Maintain Energy Levels And Avoid Overeating In One Sitting.

• **Avoid Late-Night Eating:** Avoid Eating Large Meals Or Snacks Close To Bedtime.

9. Medical Supervision:

• **Regular Monitoring:** Work Closely With Your Healthcare Team, Including A Registered Dietitian, For Regular Monitoring Of Your Nutritional Status.

- **Follow Provider Recommendations:** Adhere To Specific Guidelines Provided By Your Healthcare Team, As Individual Needs May Vary.

10. Behavioral And Emotional Support:

- **Address Emotional Eating:** If Emotional Eating Is A Concern, Consider Seeking Support From Mental Health Professionals To Develop Coping Strategies.

- **Build A Support System:** Surround Yourself With A Supportive Network Of Friends And Family To Help With Emotional And Practical Aspects Of The Pre-Surgery Period.

It's Crucial To Note That These Guidelines Are General Recommendations, And Individualized Advice From Healthcare Professionals Is Essential. The Healthcare Team, Including A Registered Dietitian Or Nutritionist, Will Assess Individual Needs And Provide Personalized Recommendations Based On Your Health Status And Specific Requirements. Adhering To Pre-Surgery Nutrition Guidelines Contributes To A Smoother Surgical Experience And Enhances The Overall Success Of Gastric Sleeve Surgery.

Mental and Emotional Preparation

Mental And Emotional Preparation Is A Crucial Aspect Of The Gastric Sleeve Journey. The Decision To Undergo Weight-Loss Surgery Represents A Significant Lifestyle Change, And Addressing Mental And Emotional Well-Being Is Essential For A Successful Outcome. Here Are Key Considerations For Mental And Emotional Preparation:

1. Educate Yourself:

• **Understand The Procedure:** Gain A Comprehensive Understanding Of The Gastric Sleeve Surgery, Including The Potential Benefits, Risks, And Post-

Operative Expectations. Knowing What To Expect Can Alleviate Anxiety And Uncertainty.

- **Attend Informational Sessions:** Attend Bariatric Seminars, Support Groups, Or Informational Sessions Provided By Healthcare Professionals To Learn From Others' Experiences And Ask Questions.

2. Set Realistic Expectations:

- **Weight-Loss Expectations:** Set Realistic Expectations For Weight Loss And Recognize That Surgery Is A Tool, Not A Guaranteed Solution. Sustainable, Long-Term Success Requires Commitment To Lifestyle Changes.

- **Physical And Emotional Changes:** Acknowledge That The Journey Involves Both Physical And Emotional Changes. Be Prepared For Adjustments In Body Image, Relationships, And Self-Perception.

3. Emotional Eating Awareness:

- **Identify Triggers:** Reflect On Emotional Eating Patterns And Identify Triggers. Recognizing Emotional Eating Behaviors Is The First Step Toward Developing Healthier Coping Mechanisms.

- **Seek Professional Support:** If Emotional Eating Is A Concern, Consider Seeking Support From Mental Health Professionals, Such As

Therapists Or Counselors, To Address Underlying Emotional Issues.

4. Build A Support System:

• **Communicate With Loved Ones:** Share Your Decision With Friends And Family. Building A Support System Can Provide Emotional Encouragement And Practical Assistance During The Pre-Operative And Post-Operative Periods.

• **Attend Support Groups:** Joining Support Groups, Whether In-Person Or Online, Allows You To Connect With Individuals Who Have Undergone Similar Experiences. Sharing Stories And Advice Can Be Valuable.

5. Address Anxiety And Fear:

• **Open Communication With Healthcare Team:** Communicate Openly With Your Healthcare Team About Any Fears Or Anxieties You May Have. They Can Provide Information, Reassurance, And Resources To Address Concerns.

• **Consider Counseling:** If Anxiety Or Fear Is Significant, Consider Seeking Counseling Or Therapy To Develop Coping Strategies And Emotional Resilience.

6. Lifestyle Changes:

• **Prepare For Lifestyle Adjustments:** Understand That

Lifestyle Changes Are An Integral Part Of The Process. Mental And Emotional Preparation Involves Accepting And Embracing These Changes, Including Dietary Modifications And Regular Exercise.

7. Create A Pre- And Post-Operative Plan:

• **Plan for Recovery:** Develop A Plan For The Pre-Operative And Post-Operative Periods. This Includes Arranging For Support During Recovery, Planning For Meal Preparation, And Scheduling Follow-Up Appointments With Healthcare Professionals.

8. Journaling and Reflection:

• **Reflect On Goals:** Journaling Can Be A Helpful Way To Reflect On Your Goals, Emotions, And Experiences Throughout The Journey. Documenting Your Thoughts Can Provide Insight Into Your Progress And Challenges.

9. Celebrate Non-Scale Victories:

• Acknowledge Achievements: Celebrate Non-Scale Victories, Such As Improvements In Energy Levels, Increased Physical Activity, Or Positive Changes In Overall Well-Being. These Achievements Are Essential For Motivation.

10. Continued Education:

• **Stay Informed:** Continue To Educate Yourself About Nutrition, Exercise, And Mental Health Throughout The Journey. Knowledge Empowers You To Make Informed Decisions And Sustain Healthy Habits.

11. Mindfulness and Relaxation Techniques:

• Incorporate Relaxation: Practice Mindfulness And Relaxation Techniques, Such As Deep Breathing Or Meditation, To Manage Stress And Stay Focused On Your Goals.

Remember That Mental And Emotional Preparation Is An Ongoing

Process, And Seeking Professional Guidance When Needed Is A Sign Of Strength. Building A Strong Foundation Of Mental And Emotional Well-Being Contributes Significantly To The Overall Success And Sustainability Of The Gastric Sleeve Journey.

Setting Realistic Expectations

Setting Realistic Expectations Is Crucial For Individuals Considering Or Undergoing Gastric Sleeve Surgery. It's Essential To Understand That While The Surgery Can Lead To Significant Weight Loss And Improvements In Health, It Is Not A Quick Fix Or A Guarantee Of A Perfect Outcome.

Here Are Key Considerations For Setting Realistic Expectations:

1. Weight Loss:

• **Realistic Goals:** Understand That Weight Loss Varies Among Individuals. While Many Experience Substantial Weight Loss In The First Year, The Rate May Slow Down Over Time.

• **Health Improvements:** Focus On Overall Health Improvements Rather Than Just The Number On The Scale. Benefits May Include Better Blood Sugar Control, Improved Mobility, And Reduced Risk Of Obesity-Related Health Conditions.

2. Lifestyle Changes:

- **Permanent Changes:** Recognize That Successful Outcomes Depend On Adopting And Maintaining Long-Term Lifestyle Changes. This Includes A Healthy, Balanced Diet, Regular Physical Activity, And Ongoing Medical Follow-Up.

- **Mindful Eating:** Embrace Mindful Eating Habits, Focusing On Quality Nutrition, Portion Control, And Listening To Hunger And Satiety Cues.

3. Body Image:

- **Realistic Body Image Expectations:** Understand That Body Image Changes Are Part Of The

Process. Loose Skin May Occur After Significant Weight Loss, And Accepting These Changes Can Be Part Of The Journey.

• **Time For Adjustment:** Give Yourself Time To Adjust To Your Changing Body. Emotional And Mental Well-Being Is A Crucial Aspect Of Post-Operative Success.

4. Emotional Changes:

• **Address Emotional Factors:** Recognize That Emotional Changes May Accompany Weight Loss. Some Individuals Experience A Range Of Emotions, Including Joy, Surprise, Or Even Challenges With Body Image.

Seeking Support From Mental Health Professionals Can Be Beneficial.

5. Dietary Adjustments:

• Gradual Dietary Progression: Understand That The Post-Operative Diet Involves A Gradual Progression From Liquids To Solid Foods. It's Essential To Follow Dietary Guidelines Provided By Healthcare Professionals For Optimal Healing And Weight Loss.

• **Potential Dietary Intolerances:** Be Aware That Some Foods May Be Better Tolerated Than Others Post-Surgery. Adjusting To New Dietary Patterns Is Part Of The Process.

6. Health Improvements:

• Focus On Non-Scale Victories: Celebrate Non-Scale Victories, Such As Improved Energy Levels, Better Sleep, Enhanced Mobility, And Reductions In Medications. These Victories Contribute To An Overall Sense Of Well-Being.

7. Setbacks and Plateaus:

• Realize Setbacks Are Normal: Recognize That Setbacks And Plateaus Are A Normal Part Of The Journey. Weight Loss May Not Always Be Linear, And It's Important To Stay Committed To Long-Term Goals.

• **Adapt Goals:** Be Flexible And Adapt Goals As Needed. The Journey May Involve Adjustments To The Initial Plan Based On Individual Responses And Health Needs.

8. Social and Relationship Dynamics:

• **Communication With Loved Ones:** Communicate Openly With Friends And Family About Your Goals And Challenges. Educate Them About The Changes You're Making And How They Can Support You.

• **Impact On Relationships:** Understand That Weight Loss May Impact Relationships, And Maintaining

Open Communication Can Help Navigate These Changes.

9. Support System:

• Build A Support System: Surround Yourself With A Supportive Network Of Friends, Family, And Healthcare Professionals. Having A Strong Support System Can Contribute To Emotional Well-Being And Success.

10. Ongoing Medical Follow-Up:

• **Regular Check-Ups:** Recognize The Importance Of Ongoing Medical Follow-Up. Regular Check-Ups Help Monitor Progress, Address Concerns, And Make Necessary Adjustments To The Treatment Plan.

By Setting Realistic Expectations And Embracing The Holistic Nature Of The Gastric Sleeve Journey, Individuals Can Approach The Process With A Positive Mindset, Resilience, And A Greater Likelihood Of Achieving Long-Term Success. Regular Communication With Healthcare Professionals And Support From Loved Ones Play Pivotal Roles In Navigating The Challenges And Triumphs Along The Way.

CHAPTER THREE
Important Post-Surgery Care Tips

Post-Surgery Care Is Crucial For The Successful Recovery And Long-Term Success Of Gastric Sleeve Surgery. Here Are Important Post-Surgery Care Tips To Follow:

1. Follow Medical Advice:

- **Adhere To Guidelines:** Strictly Follow The Post-Operative Guidelines Provided By Your Healthcare Team, Including Dietary Recommendations, Activity Restrictions, And Medication Instructions.

- **Attend Follow-Up Appointments:** Schedule And Attend All Follow-Up

Appointments With Your Surgeon And Healthcare Team For Regular Monitoring And Adjustments To Your Care Plan.

2. Dietary Guidelines:

• **Progress Gradually:** Adhere To The Gradual Dietary Progression Recommended By Your Healthcare Team. Start With Clear Liquids, Progress To Pureed And Soft Foods, And Then Transition To A Balanced Solid Food Diet.

• **Hydration:** Stay Well-Hydrated By Sipping Water Throughout The Day. Avoid Drinking With Meals To Prevent Overloading Your Stomach.

• **Protein Intake:** Prioritize Protein-Rich Foods To Support Healing, Muscle Preservation, And Overall Nutrition.

• Avoid High-Calorie, Low-Nutrient Foods: Limit Intake Of Sugary And High-Fat Foods. Focus On Nutrient-Dense Options For Optimal Health.

3. Physical Activity:

• **Gradual Exercise:** Gradually Incorporate Light Physical Activity Into Your Routine As Advised By Your Healthcare Team. Start With Short Walks And Progressively Increase Intensity.

• **Follow Activity Restrictions:** Adhere To Any Activity Restrictions

Provided By Your Surgeon, Especially During The Initial Weeks Of Recovery.

4. Medication Management:

- **Take Prescribed Medications:** Take All Prescribed Medications As Directed By Your Healthcare Provider, Including Pain Medications And Any Recommended Supplements.

- **Avoid Certain Medications:** Avoid Non-Steroidal Anti-Inflammatory Drugs (Nsaids) And Aspirin Unless Specifically Approved By Your Surgeon, As They May Increase The Risk Of Complications.

5. Hygiene and Wound Care:

• **Follow Wound Care Instructions**: If You Have Incisions, Follow The Wound Care Instructions Provided By Your Surgeon. Keep The Incision Area Clean And Dry.

• **Watch For Signs Of Infection:** Monitor For Signs Of Infection, Such As Increased Redness, Swelling, Or Discharge From The Incision Site. Report Any Concerns To Your Healthcare Provider Promptly.

6. Listen To Your Body:

• **Recognize Satiety:** Pay Attention To Feelings Of Fullness And Stop Eating When You Feel Satisfied. Overeating

Can Lead To Discomfort And Complications.

• **Rest And Recovery:** Ensure You Get Adequate Rest And Sleep To Support The Healing Process. Avoid Strenuous Activities During The Initial Recovery Period.

7. Behavioral and Emotional Support:

• **Seek Support:** If Needed, Consider Seeking Support From Mental Health Professionals Or Support Groups To Address Emotional And Behavioral Aspects Of The Post-Operative Period.

• **Address Emotional Eating:** Continue To Work On Identifying And

Addressing Emotional Eating Triggers And Patterns.

8. Stay Hydrated:

• **Water Intake:** Drink Water Regularly To Stay Hydrated. Proper Hydration Supports Overall Health and Aids in Digestion.

9. Vitamin and Mineral Supplements:

• **Take As Prescribed:** If Prescribed, Take Vitamin And Mineral Supplements As Directed To Prevent Deficiencies. Regular Monitoring Of Nutrient Levels May Be Necessary.

10. Gradual Return To Normal Activities:

• **Return to Work:** Gradually Ease Back Into Work And Daily Activities Based On Your Surgeon's Recommendations.

• **Resume Exercise:** As Your Surgeon Permits, Resume Regular Exercise And Physical Activities Gradually.

11. Celebrate Milestones:

• **Acknowledge Achievements:** Celebrate Non-Scale Victories And Milestones In Your Weight Loss Journey. Recognize Gains In Energy Levels, Movement, And Overall Well-Being.

12. Ongoing Monitoring:

- **Regular Check-Ups:** Continue Regular Check-Ups With Your Healthcare Team To Monitor Progress, Address Any Concerns, And Ensure Ongoing Support.

Remember, Each Individual's Recovery Process Is Unique, And It's Important To Communicate Openly With Your Healthcare Team. If You Experience Any Unusual Symptoms, Complications, Or Have Concerns, Contact Your Healthcare Provider Promptly. Following These Post-Surgery Care Tips Will Contribute To A Smoother Recovery And Enhance Your Chances Of Achieving Long-Term Success With Gastric Sleeve Surgery.

Phase of Clear Liquid Diet

The Clear Liquid Diet Is A Distinct Phase In The Postoperative Treatment For Patients Who Have Had Gastric Sleeve Surgery. During The Early Postoperative Period, This Phase Has Multiple Functions Such As Preventing Dehydration, Reducing Strain On The Healing Stomach, And Aiding In The Shift To A More Diverse Diet. Key Components Of The Clear Liquid Diet Phase Are Outlined Below:

Clear Liquid Diet Purpose:

1. Encourage Hydration: Consuming Clear Liquids Is Crucial For Maintaining Hydration, Particularly During The Initial Phases Of Recovery

When Normal Food Consumption Is Limited.

2. Reduce Stomach Strain: Clear Liquids Are Easier For The Stomach To Digest, Alleviating Pressure On The Recovering Surgical Area.

3. Stomach Tolerance Monitoring: The Transparent Liquid Phase Enables Healthcare Providers To Assess The Stomach's Ability To Handle Fluids And Detect Any Urgent Issues.

Accepted Transparent Beverages:

• Water Is Essential For Maintaining Hydration.

- Clear Broths Are Produced From Poultry Or Vegetables Without Any Solid Components.

- Sugar-Free Jello: Gelatin Treats Made Without Additional Sugar.

- Sugar-Free Popsicles: Frozen Treats Without Added Sugar Can Help With Hydration.

- Clear Fruit Juices: Thinned, Sugar-Free Fruit Juices Without Pulp.

- Decaffeinated Tea Or Coffee Can Be Eaten Without Cream Or Sugar.

- Transparent Protein Beverages: Certain Transparent Protein Drinks May Be Advised By Healthcare Providers.

Guidelines and Considerations:

• **Small Sips:** Consume Drinks In Small Amounts Periodically Throughout The Day Instead Of Consuming Huge Quantities At Once.

• Consume Liquids At A Steady Pace To Avoid Overwhelming The Stomach.

• Avoid Carbonated Beverages To Reduce Gas And Bloating During This Phase.

• **Clear Liquids Only;** Colored Or Opaque Liquids Are Not Allowed. Avoid Beverages That Are Colorful Or Opaque, As They May Contain Particles That Might Cause Irritation To The Stomach.

- **Supplement Intake:** Follow Healthcare Professionals' Instructions And Consume Any Prescribed Vitamin Or Mineral Supplements During This Phase.

Length of Time:

The Transparent Liquid Phase Often Only Lasts For A Short Duration, Usually During The Initial Days Following Surgery. The Time May Vary Depending On Individual Progress And Advice From Healthcare Providers.

Progress to the Following Stage:

Once The Clear Liquid Phase Is Completed, Individuals Will Advance Through Subsequent Stages Of The Postoperative Diet, Such As Full

Liquids, Pureed Foods, Soft Foods, And Finally A Regular Diet. Healthcare Specialists Usually Oversee The Transfer Process, Considering Each Person's Tolerance And Healing Progress.

It Is Essential To Follow The Healthcare Team's Advice Carefully During The Clear Liquid Phase And As You Advance Through The Postoperative Diet. Regular Communication With Healthcare Specialists, Good Hydration, And Following Dietary Instructions Lead To A Smooth Recovery After Gastric Sleeve Surgery.

Switching To Pureed Foods

Transitioning To Pureed Foods Is An Essential Phase In The Postoperative Dietary Progression After Gastric Sleeve Surgery. This Period Usually Follows The Clear Liquid Diet Phase And Before The Introduction Of Solid Foods. Here Are Essential Instructions For Shifting To Pureed Foods:

Purpose of the Pureed Food Phase:

• **Enhance Healing:** Pureed Foods Aid With Digestion, Reducing Strain On The Healing Surgical Area.

• Gradual Introduction Of Texture Involves Introducing Pureed Foods To Help The Stomach Adjust To A More

Diverse Texture, As Part Of The Journey Towards Solid Foods.

Authorized Pureed Foods:

1. Low-Fat Proteins: Pureed Poultry That Has Been Cooked, Soft Fish & Tofu

2. Vegetables:

• Vegetables Including Carrots, Peas, And Sweet Potatoes That Are Thoroughly Cooked And Mashed

3. Fruits: Soft, Ripe Fruits Such As Bananas And Avocados

4. Cereals: Pureed Cooked Grains like Rice or Quinoa

5. Dairy: Low-Fat Or Fat-Free Plain Yogurt

Preparation Instructions:

• Blend or Puree by Using a Blender, Food Processor, Or Immersion Blender To Create A Smooth Consistency.

• Moisten With Broth: Add A Small Quantity Of Low-Sodium Broth Or Water Until Reaching The Desired Consistency.

• Avoid Using Potent Seasonings And Spices During The Pureed Meal Period To Prevent Gastrointestinal Irritation.

• Check The Consistency Of The Pureed Foods To Ensure They Are

Smooth And Free Of Lumps For Easier Digestion.

Portion Control and Eating Behavior:

• Start With Tiny Portions And Consume Your Food Gradually. The Stomach Has A Finite Capacity, And Consuming An Excessive Amount Of Food Might Cause Pain.

• Attend To Signals Of Hunger And Fullness. Cease Eating When You Are Satiated And Refrain From Eating Quickly.

• Stay Hydrated By Drinking Water Between Meals.

Frequency and Advancement:

• Gradually Increase The Frequency Of Pureed Meals While Ensuring Consistent Hydration.

• **Transition To Solid Foods:** The Shift To Solid Foods Is Usually Overseen By Healthcare Specialists According To Each Person's Advancement And Ability To Tolerate Them. Adhere Strictly To Their Recommendations.

Extra Suggestions:

• Seek Advice From Healthcare Professionals: If You Are Uncertain About Certain Foods Or Serving Sizes, Check With Your Healthcare Team Or

A Registered Dietitian For Tailored Advice.

• Ensure Sufficient Nutrient Intake By Maintaining A Balanced Diet While Moving To Pureed Meals.

• Prioritize Nutrient-Dense Foods And Avoid Consuming High-Calorie, Low-Nutrient Choices.

• Gradually Reintroduce Textured Foods As Tolerated To Prepare For The Transition To Solid Foods.

Following These Rules And Maintaining Regular Communication With Healthcare Providers Facilitates A Seamless Transition To The Pureed Food Stage Post Gastric Sleeve Surgery. Individual Outcomes Can

Differ, Thus It Is Crucial To Adhere To The Precise Guidelines Given By The Healthcare Staff To Enhance The Recovery Process.

CHAPTER FOUR
Developing Purees with High Nutritional Value

It Is Crucial To Make Nutrient-Dense Purees During The Postoperative Period, Particularly When Moving To Pureed Foods Following Gastric Sleeve Surgery. The Purees Are Designed To Deliver Vital Nutrients To Support Healing And Recuperation Without Causing Stomach Discomfort. Here Are Some Suggestions For Nutrient-Dense Purees:

1. High-Protein Purees:

• Chicken or Turkey Puree:

• Cooked and Shredded Poultry

- Blend With A Little Quantity Of Low-Sodium Chicken Broth Until It Becomes Smooth.

- Season With A Dash Of Salt And Pepper

- **Fish Puree:**

  - Cooked and Shredded Tender Fish, Like Tilapia Or Sole
  - Puree with A Small Amount Of Lemon Juice And A Hint Of Olive Oil.

- **Tofu Puree:**

- Silken Tofu Mixed With Sautéed Veggies and A Bit Of Vegetable Broth

2. Vegetable Purees:

- Carrot and Ginger Puree:
- Carrots That Have Been Cooked, Mashed, And Flavored With A Touch Of Fresh Ginger
- Season with a Dash of Salt
- Pea and Mint Puree:
- Peas That Have Been Cooked And Mixed With Fresh Mint Leaves

- Include A Modest Quantity Of Vegetable Broth To Adjust The Consistency

• Butternut Squash Puree:

- Roasted and Mashed Butternut Squash

Season with a Hint of Nutmeg and a Touch of Salt

3. Fruit Purees:

- Banana And Avocado Puree:
- Blend Ripe Banana And Avocado Till Smooth.
- Add Honey For Sweetness, If Preferred.

Applesauce:

- Cooked and Blended Apples with a Dash Of Cinnamon
- Make Sure The Apples Are Tender To Facilitate Mixing.

4. Grain and Legume Purees:

• Quinoa and Vegetable Puree:

• Quinoa Cooked and Mixed With Pureed Vegetables Like Zucchini Or Spinach

• Include A Small Amount Of Vegetable Broth To Achieve A Smoother Consistency

• **Lentil Puree:**

• Sautéed Lentils Mixed With Sautéed Veggies And A Hint Of Vegetable Broth

• Season With Cumin And Coriander To Enhance The Taste.

5. Dairy and Yogurt Purees:

• **Greek Yogurt Mixed With A Berry Puree:**

• Greek Yogurt Mixed With A Variety Of Fruit Such As Strawberries, Blueberries, And Raspberries.

• Drizzle With Honey To Sweeten, If Preferred.

• **Cottage Cheese With Pineapple Puree:**

• Cottage Cheese Mixed With Fresh Or Canned Pineapple Pieces

• Make Sure The Pineapple Is Thoroughly Drained To Manage Its Texture.

Guidelines for Making Nutrient-Dense Purees:

1. Choose Fresh, Complete Foods To Enhance The Nutritional Value.

2. Incorporate A Range Of Colors:
Various Colors In Fruits And Vegetables Indicate Diverse Nutrient Compositions. Strive For A Diverse Array Of Colors To Guarantee A Wide Variety Of Nutrients.

3. Season Thoughtfully: Utilize Herbs And Spices To Enrich Flavors Without Introducing Superfluous Calories Or Irritants. Refrain From Using Too Much Salt And Spicy Flavors.

4. Include Healthy Fats Such As Olive Oil, Avocado, Or Almonds To Enhance Nutritional Content And Supply Necessary Fatty Acids.

5. Consider Nutrient Supplements: If Recommended By Healthcare

Specialists, Think About Adding Vitamin And Mineral Supplements To Fulfill Dietary Requirements.

6. Modify The Consistency And Texture Of Purees According To Each Person's Tolerance And Recovery Stage. Some Individuals May Choose Smoother Textures At First.

7. Stay Hydrated By Drinking Water between Meals and With Pureed Foods.

Seek Advice From Your Healthcare Team Or A Certified Dietitian For Tailored Assistance According To Your Individual Nutritional Requirements And Advancement. Customizing Purees To Meet Specific Preferences

And Dietary Needs Is Essential For A Healthy And Satisfying Recuperation Following Gastric Sleeve Surgery.

Phase of Soft Food

The Soft Food Phase Is An Important Stage In The Postoperative Dietary Progression Following Gastric Sleeve Surgery. This Phase Usually Comes After The Pureed Food Stage And Before Solid Meals Are Reintroduced. The Soft Food Phase Permits A Wider Range Of Textures While Maintaining Easy Digestibility Of The Foods. Below Are Instructions And Suggestions For The Soft Food Stage:

Purpose of the Soft Food Phase:

• Gradual Introduction Of Texture Involves Transitioning From Pureed To Solid Foods By Incorporating Soft Foods, Which Assist The Stomach In Adjusting To A Diverse Texture.

• Opt For Nutrient-Dense Soft Meals To Provide Critical Nutrients For The Body's Healing And Recovery.

Accepted Pureed Foods:

1. Proteins

Soft-Cooked Poultry: Well-Cooked Shredded or Diced Poultry That Is Tender.

Fish: Soft and Flaky Fish Such As Tilapia or Salmon.

Eggs: Scrambled Or Soft-Boiled Eggs.

2. Vegetables:

Mashed Sweet Potatoes: Mashed Sweet Potatoes Cooked With Butter Or Olive Oil.

Steamed Or Softly Cooked Vegetables: Carrots, Broccoli, And Green Beans Boiled Until Tender.

Avocado: Avocado That Is Sliced Or Mashed.

3. Fruits:

Unsweetened Applesauce.

Canned Or Cooked Fruits:

• Fruit Such As Peaches, Pears, Or Berries That Have Been Tenderized Through The Process Of Cooking.

4. Dairy:

Greek Yogurt: Low-Fat or Fat-Free Greek Yogurt.

Cottage Cheese: Soft and Well-Drained Cottage Cheese.

5. Cereals and Pulses:

Cooked Quinoa: Cooked Quinoa Till Tender.

Lentils:

• Tender and Well-Prepared Lentils.

Soft Food Phase Guidelines:

1. Control The Amount Of Food Consumed:

• Continue Consuming Modest, Regular Meals To Prevent Overwhelming The Stomach.

• Pay Attention To Your Body's Hunger And Fullness Signals, And Stop Eating When You Feel Satisfied.

2. Chew Meticulously:

• Chew Soft Meals Completely To Assist In Digestion And Avoid Discomfort.

3. Avoid Foods That Are Difficult To Chew Or Have A Fibrous Texture.

Avoid Consuming Hard Meats, Fibrous Vegetables, And Foods That May Be Difficult To Digest.

4. Keep Yourself Well-Hydrated.

• Continue To Prioritize Hydration By Intermittently Drinking Water Throughout The Day.

5. Avoid Fizzy Drinks.

• Avoid Or Limit Fizzy Beverages To Prevent Gas And Discomfort.

6. Monitor For Tolerance.

• Observe Your Body's Responses To Various Foods And Modify Your Diet According To Your Personal Tolerance.

7. Progressive Incorporation of Textures:

• If You Feel At Ease, You May Want To Start Incorporating Slightly More Textured Meals To Help With The Gradual Shift To Solid Foods.

8. Regular Monitoring:

• Continue Routine Appointments With Healthcare Providers To Track Improvement, Discuss Any Issues, And Receive Consistent Assistance.

Soft Food Meal Suggestions:

1. Chicken and Vegetable Stir-Fry:

• Tender Chicken With Thoroughly Cooked Veggies.

Season With Gentle Spices And Soy Sauce.

2. Avocado and Tuna Salad Mash:

• Mixture Of Mashed Avocado And Canned Tuna.

• Season With Lemon Juice And Salt.

3. Spinach Scrambled Eggs:

• Soft Scrambled Eggs With Sautéed Spinach.

4. Tender Turkey And Cheese Roll-Ups:

• Turkey Deli Meat Wrapped Around Soft Cheese.

5. Sweet Potato and Chicken Casserole with Mashed Sweet Potatoes.

• Layers Of Mashed Sweet Potato And Shredded Chicken Cooked Until Warm.

6. Greek Yogurt Parfait:

• Alternate Layers Of Greek Yogurt With Tender Fruits Such As Berries.

7. Quinoa and Vegetable Bowl:

• Quinoa Combined With Tender-Cooked Veggies.

Following The Suggestions And Slowly Incorporating A Range Of Nutrient-Dense Soft Foods Aids In A Successful Recovery And Readies The Digestive System For Transitioning Back To A

Normal Diet. Always Seek Guidance From Healthcare Specialists Or A Trained Dietician For Tailored Counsel According To Your Specific Requirements And Development.

CHAPTER FIVE
Constructing a Well-Balanced Diet

Establishing A Well-Rounded Diet Is Crucial For Maintaining Good Health And Wellness, Especially Following Gastric Sleeve Surgery. The Procedure Decreases The Stomach's Size, Reducing Its Capacity, And Requires Careful Monitoring Of Nutrient Intake. Key Elements For Creating A Well-Rounded Diet Post Gastric Sleeve Surgery:

1. Emphasize Protein Consumption.

Protein Is Essential For Promoting Healing, Preserving Muscle Mass, And Sustaining General Health. It Is Crucial, Particularly Following Surgery.

- **Sources:** Incorporate Lean Protein Sources Such Poultry, Fish, Lean Meats, Eggs, Tofu, And Low-Fat Dairy Products.

- **Supplementation:** Use Protein Shakes or Powders As Recommended By Healthcare Professionals, If Necessary.

2. Include A Diverse Selection Of Vegetables.

- **Nutrient Density:** Vegetables Include High Levels Of Vitamins, Minerals, And Fiber, With Low Calorie Content.

- Incorporate A Diverse Selection Of Colorful Veggies To Guarantee A Wide Array Of Nutrients.

3. Consume Fruits In Moderation:

• Fruits Are Nutrient-Dense As They Include Vital Vitamins, Minerals, And Antioxidants.

• Practice Moderation with Sugar by Opting For Whole Fruits Instead Of Fruit Juices and Restricting Consumption of High-Sugar Fruits.

4. Choose Whole Grains.

• Whole Grains Offer Fiber, Vitamins, and Minerals. Select Options Such As Quinoa, Brown Rice, Oats, And Whole Wheat.

• Practice Portion Control by Being Aware Of Serving Sizes to Prevent Consuming Too Many Calories.

5. Include Nutritious Fats:

• Incorporate Sources Of Healthy Fats Including Avocados, Nuts, Seeds, And Olive Oil.

• Practice Moderation by Being Cautious Of Portion Sizes to Manage Calorie Consumption, Notwithstanding the Significance of Healthy Fats.

6. Select Low-Fat Dairy Products.

• Low-Fat Or Fat-Free Dairy Products Are A Good Source Of Vital Calcium And Protein.

• If You Are Lactose Intolerant, You Should Opt For Lactose-Free Alternatives Or Calcium Supplements.

7. Stay Properly Hydrated.

• Hydrate Yourself Adequately By Drinking Water Consistently Throughout The Day. Sufficient Hydration Promotes Digestion And Overall Well-Being.

• Reduce Consumption Of Caloric Liquids: Limit Intake Of Sugary Drinks, Sodas, And High-Calorie Beverages.

8. Mindful Eating

• Chew Food Completely To Assist Digestion, Particularly Crucial Following Gastric Sleeve Surgery.

• Attend To Hunger And Fullness Signals: Be Mindful Of Indicators

Indicating Hunger And Fullness. Cease Eating Until You Are Satisfied.

9. Choose Your Supplements Wisely.

• Take Vitamin And Mineral Supplements As Advised By Healthcare Professionals To Prevent Deficiencies Based On Individual Requirements.

• Gastric Sleeve Surgery Can Affect The Absorption Of Vitamin B12 And Iron, Potentially Requiring Supplements.

10. Avoid Processed And High-Calorie Foods.

• Opt For Nutrient-Dense Foods Instead Of Processed And High-Calorie Ones To Improve Nutritional Intake.

• Practice Moderation When Consuming Treats To Uphold A Balanced Diet While Still Achieving Health Objectives.

11. Routine Follow-Up And Monitoring:

• **Health Check-Ups:** Regularly See Healthcare Professionals, Such As A Nutritionist, To Assess Nutritional Status And Make Necessary Adjustments To The Diet.

• **Laboratory Analysis:** Regular Lab Testing Can Assist In Detecting And Resolving Any Vitamin Shortages.

12. Take Into Account Individual Preferences And Tolerances.

• Personalized Approach: Customize Your Diet To Align With Your Preferences, Cultural Factors, And Individual Tolerances.

• Experiment With Different Cuisines To Determine The Most Suitable Options For You While Ensuring Nutritional Requirements Are Met.

13. Timing of Meals:

• Consistently Consume Balanced Meals And Snacks To Sustain Energy Levels And Avoid Extreme Hunger.

Avoid Eating Late At Night To Improve Digestion And Sleep Quality.

14. Exercise:

• Gradually Reintroduce And Enhance Physical Activity As Advised By Healthcare Professionals.

• Incorporate Strength Training Workouts To Maintain And Increase Muscle Mass.

To Establish A Well-Rounded Diet Following Gastric Sleeve Surgery, One Must Meticulously Plan, Focus On Nutrient Consumption, And Consistently Evaluate Nutritional Levels. Consulting With Healthcare Specialists, Such As A Qualified Dietitian, Is Essential For Tailored Guidance And Assistance Due To Individual Variations In Needs. An

Optimal And Healthy Diet Is Crucial For Enhancing The Recovery Process And Sustaining Long-Term Health.

Significance of Protein Consumption

Protein Consumption Is Crucial, Particularly Following Gastric Sleeve Surgery. Protein Has Various Essential Functions In Promoting General Well-Being, Especially After Surgery. Here Are Some Arguments Emphasizing The Need Of Protein Consumption Following Gastric Sleeve Surgery:

1. Healing and Recovery of Tissues:

• Protein Is Vital For Cell Repair And Regeneration, Which Is Critical For The Healing Process Post-Surgery.

Proper Protein Consumption Promotes Effective Wound Healing And Decreases The Likelihood Of Problems From Surgical Incisions.

2. Maintaining Muscle Mass:

• **Lean Muscle Preservation:** Protein Is Essential For Maintaining Lean Muscle Mass. Following Gastric Sleeve Surgery, It Is Essential To Prioritize The Preservation Of Muscle Mass To Support Metabolic Well-Being And General Physical Strength.

• **Muscle Wasting Prevention:** Sufficient Protein Consumption Can Prevent Muscle Wasting, A Condition That May Arise During Weight

Reduction Or Decreased Caloric Intake.

3. Immune System Function:

• Proteins Are Essential For Producing Antibodies And Components Of The Immune System, Which Enhance Immunological Response.

• Proper Diet, Which Includes Sufficient Protein Consumption, Enhances Immune Function And Decreases The Likelihood Of Infections During The Healing Phase.

4. Transporting and Storing Nutrients:

• Proteins Aid in the Transportation Of Vital Elements Such As Vitamins And Minerals Throughout The Body.

• **Nutrient Storage:** Certain Proteins Are Responsible For Storing Essential Nutrients To Maintain A Consistent Supply For Different Body Processes.

5. Regulation of Hormones:

• Proteins Have A Role In Synthesizing Hormones That Control Several Physiological Functions Such As Metabolism And Energy Balance.

• Protein Intake Can Assist In Controlling Blood Sugar Levels,

Especially Crucial For Persons With A History Of Obesity And Metabolic Disorders.

6. Fullness and Weight Control:

• Protein-Rich Foods Help Create A Sense Of Fullness And Satiety, Which Can Help Regulate Appetite And Support Weight Control.

• The Body Requires More Energy To Digest And Metabolize Protein Than Fats And Carbs, Resulting In A Greater Calorie-Burning Effect.

7. Nutrient-Rich Choice:

• Protein-Rich Foods Are Often Nutrient-Dense Due To The Presence Of Vital Vitamins And Minerals.

8. Following Dietary Guidelines:

• After Gastric Sleeve Surgery, Healthcare Providers Stress The Significance Of Achieving Protein Goals As Part Of The Postoperative Dietary Requirements.

• **Enhancing Dietary Advancement:** Sufficient Protein Consumption Aids In The Shift From Liquid To Pureed To Solid Diets, Guaranteeing The Body Obtains Vital Nutrients During Each Phase Of Recuperation.

9. Hair and Nail Health:

• **Keratin Synthesis:** Proteins, Especially Keratin, Are Essential For The Well-Being And Durability Of Hair And Nails. Postoperative Food

Decisions Can Affect The Health Of These Structures.

10. Personalized Requirements:

Individuals Have Varying Protein Requirements, And Healthcare Professionals Can Offer Individualized Recommendations Considering Aspects Like Weight, Exercise Level, And Overall Health.

Strategies for Achieving Protein Targets Post Gastric Sleeve Surgery:

• Choose Lean Protein Sources Such Poultry, Fish, Lean Meats, Tofu, And Low-Fat Dairy.

• Spread Out Protein Intake Evenly By Consuming It At Every Meal And Snack

To Maintain A Steady Supply Throughout The Day.

• If Dietary Protein Intake Is Difficult, Healthcare Providers May Suggest Protein Supplements Or Smoothies To Help Reach Daily Targets.

• Monitor Protein Consumption To Ensure It Aligns With Individual Protein Objectives By Tracking And Adjusting Food Choices Accordingly.

• Consult A Trained Dietitian To Create A Customized Dietary Plan That Fulfills Protein Requirements, Taking Into Account Personal Preferences And Tolerances.

Ensuring Sufficient Protein Consumption Is A Crucial Aspect Of

The Postoperative Care Regimen For Those Who Have Had Gastric Sleeve Surgery. It Aids In Healing, Muscular Retention, And Overall Well-Being Throughout The Recovery Phase. Consistent Interaction With Medical Specialists And Following Dietary Recommendations Are Key Factors In A Successful Recovery After Surgery.

Hydration and Nutritional Supplements

Hydration And Nutritional Supplements Are Vital Components Of Postoperative Care, Particularly Following Gastric Sleeve Surgery. These Components Are Crucial For Aiding Recovery, Avoiding Problems, And Maintaining Peak Health.

Examining The Significance Of Staying Hydrated And Taking Nutritional Supplements After Gastric Sleeve Surgery:

Moisture:

1. Facilitates The Process Of Healing: Proper Hydration Is Crucial For The Healing Process. It Aids In Cellular Repair And Regeneration, Promoting The Recovery Of Tissues And Organs.

2. Prevents Desiccation: Post-Surgery, Dehydration Risk May Arise From Causes Such As Decreased Oral Intake, Alterations In Fluid Balance, And Heightened Fluid Losses During The Initial Recovery Phase.

3.   Facilitates   Digestion: Proper Hydration Facilitates Digestion, Promoting Efficient Nutrition Absorption And Reducing The Risk Of Issues Like Constipation.

4. Reduces Feelings Of Nausea And Tiredness. Hydration Decreases Postoperative Symptoms Such As Nausea And Exhaustion, Enhancing Overall Comfort And Well-Being.

5.   Regulates   Electrolyte   Levels: Electrolyte Homeostasis Is Essential For Multiple Physiological Functions. Proper Hydration Helps Maintain Electrolyte Balance, Reducing Potential Consequences From Imbalances.

6. Promotes Frequent Urination. Adequate Hydration Promotes Frequent Urine, Aiding In The Removal Of Waste Products From The Body And Maintaining Kidney Function.

7. Hydration Guidelines: Stay Hydrated By Drinking Water Consistently Throughout The Day.

•   Avoid Consuming Excessive Quantities At Once To Prevent Discomfort.

•   Avoid Consuming Excessive Amounts Of Caffeinated And Sugary Drinks.

Dietary Supplements:

1. Prevents Lack Of Essential Nutrients:

• Gastric Sleeve Surgery Might Affect The Absorption Of Nutrients. Nutritional Supplements Aid In Preventing Shortages Of Vital Vitamins And Minerals.

2. Facilitates The Process Of Healing:

• Specific Nutrients Like Vitamin C And Zinc Are Essential For The Process Of Wound Healing. Supplements Can Help Maintain Sufficient Levels During The Healing Period.

3. Meets Precise Nutritional Requirements.

• Healthcare Specialists May Suggest Certain Supplements, Including Iron, Vitamin B12, Calcium, Based On Individual Needs.

4. Regulates Nutrient Consumption:

• Nutritional Supplements Aid In Maintaining A Balanced Nutritional Intake, Particularly When Dietary Restrictions Or Tolerances Restrict The Range Of Foods Eaten.

5. Routine Surveillance:

• Regularly Monitoring Vitamin Levels Via Blood Testing Enables Healthcare

Practitioners To Modify Supplement Dosages As Necessary.

6. Nutritional Supplements Guidelines: Follow The Specified Supplement Regimen Provided By Healthcare Providers.

• Select Premium Supplements To Guarantee Maximum Absorption.

• Spread Out The Intake Of Supplements Throughout The Day To Improve Absorption.

Guidelines for Staying Hydrated and Consuming Nutritional Supplements:

1. Organized Timetable:

• Create A Systematic Timetable For Consuming Fluids And Supplements Over The Day.

2. Observe The Color Of Your Urine.

• Monitor Urine Color As A Broad Measure Of Hydration Status. A Pale Yellow Color Usually Indicates Sufficient Hydration.

3. Collaborate With Healthcare Professionals.

• Collaborate Closely With Healthcare Specialists, Such As Dietitians, To

Assess Individual Hydration Needs And Supplement Requirements.

4. Progressive Implementation of Supplements:

• Gradually Introduce Dietary Supplements, Particularly During The Early Postoperative Phase, To Evaluate Tolerance.

5. Pay Attention To Your Body's Signals.

• Monitor Your Body's Reaction To Hydration And Supplements Closely, And Inform Your Healthcare Staff Of Any Issues Or Negative Effects.

6. Select Suitable Forms:

• Choose Vitamins That Are Easily Tolerated, Including Liquid Or Chewable Formulations, Particularly In The Initial Phases Of Recuperation.

7. Regular Monitoring:

• Attend Scheduled Follow-Up Sessions With Healthcare Providers To Evaluate Nutritional Status, Make Required Modifications, And Discuss Any Issues.

Hydration And Nutritional Supplements Are Essential Parts Of The Postoperative Care Regimen Following Gastric Sleeve Surgery. Adhering To Rules, Maintaining Hydration, And Adhering To

Prescribed Supplements Aid In A Speedier Recovery, Reduce Problems, And Promote Long-Term Health And Well-Being.

CHAPTER SIX
Dietary Planning and Portion Management

Meal Planning And Portion Management Are Essential Components Of Postoperative Care Following Gastric Sleeve Surgery. These Techniques Aid Individuals In Regulating Their Dietary Consumption, Promoting Healing, And Attaining And Sustaining A Healthy Weight. Below Are Instructions For Efficient Meal Preparation And Portion Management Following Gastric Sleeve Surgery:

Menu Organization:

1. Well-Rounded Meals:

• Plan Meals That Incorporate A Mix Of Protein, Veggies, Fruits, And Whole Grains To Guarantee A Diverse Range Of Vital Nutrients.

2. Consistent Eating Schedule:

• Strive For Consistent Meals And Snacks Throughout The Day To Maintain A Continuous Flow Of Nutrients And Avoid Extreme Hunger.

3. Emphasis on Protein:

• Emphasize Protein In Every Meal To Aid In Healing, Preserve Muscle Mass, And Enhance Feelings Of Fullness.

4. Foods Rich in Nutrients:

• Incorporate Nutrient-Dense Foods Like Vegetables, Fruits, Lean Meats, And Whole Grains To Optimize Nutritional Consumption.

5. Moisture:

• Integrate Water Into Your Meals And Drink It Gradually Throughout The Day To Stay Hydrated. Restrict High-Calorie Drinks.

6. Gradual Food Introduction:

• Gradually Reintroduce A Variety Of Foods Based On Individual Tolerance And Healthcare Professional Suggestions.

7. Mindful Eating:

• Practice Mindful Eating By Savoring Each Bite, Chewing Properly, And Paying Attention To Hunger And Fullness Signs.

8. Consult With A Dietitian:

• Work With A Licensed Dietitian To Establish Tailored Meal Plans That Fit Individual Nutritional Needs, Preferences, And Dietary Tolerances.

Portion Control:

1. Small, Frequent Meals:

• Opt For Smaller, More Frequent Meals To Avoid Overwhelming The Lower Stomach Capacity. Aim For

Roughly Five To Six Modest Meals Per Day.

2. Use Smaller Plates And Utensils:

• Choose Smaller Plates And Utensils To Provide The Idea Of Greater Amounts While Controlling Real Intake.

3. Protein First:

• Consume Protein-Rich Foods First During Meals To Prioritize Essential Nutrients.

4. Avoid Grazing:

• Limit Continuous Snacking Or Grazing Between Meals To Prevent Excessive Calorie Intake.

5. Listen To Your Body:

• Pay Attention To Your Body's Signals Of Hunger And Fullness. Stop Eating When Satisfied To Prevent Discomfort.

6. Limit Liquid Intake During Meals:

• Avoid Drinking Large Amounts Of Liquids During Meals, As This Can Contribute To Feelings Of Fullness And Potentially Lead To Discomfort.

7. Pre-Portion Snacks:

• Pre-Portion Snacks In Advance To Avoid Mindless Eating And Control Calorie Intake.

8. Use Food Logs:

• Keep A Food Log Or Use A Tracking App To Monitor Daily Food Intake And Ensure Adherence To Dietary Guidelines.

Sample Meal Plan:

Here's A Sample Meal Plan To Illustrate The Principles Of Meal Planning And Portion Control:

Breakfast:

• Scrambled Eggs with Spinach And Feta Cheese

• Small Serving of Greek Yogurt

Snack:

• Sliced Apple with a Tablespoon Of Almond Butter

Lunch:

• Grilled Chicken Salad with Mixed Greens, Cherry Tomatoes, and Vinaigrette Dressing

Snack:

• Cottage Cheese with Pineapple Chunks

Dinner:

• Baked Fish Fillet with Roasted Vegetables (Zucchini, Bell Peppers, and Carrots)

• Quinoa or Brown Rice

Snack:

• **Small Handful of Nuts**

Tips for Success:

1. Preparation Is Key:

Plan Meals And Snacks In Advance To Avoid Impulsive Choices.

2. Vary Your Choices:

• Include A Variety Of Foods To Ensure A Well-Rounded Nutritional Profile.

3. Introduce New Foods Gradually:

• Gradually Reintroduce New Foods To Assess Tolerance And Identify Any Potential Triggers.

4. Stay Consistent:

• Aim For Consistency In Meal Timing And Portion Sizes To Establish A Routine.

5. Seek Professional Guidance:

• Consult With Healthcare Professionals, Including A Dietitian, For Personalized Guidance And Adjustments To Your Meal Plan.

By Incorporating These Meal Planning And Portion Control Strategies, Individuals Can Optimize Their Nutrition, Support The Recovery Process, And Maintain A Healthy Weight After Gastric Sleeve Surgery. Regular Communication With Healthcare Professionals And

Adherence To Dietary Guidelines Contribute To Long-Term Success And Well-Being.

Overcoming Challenges

Overcoming Challenges After Gastric Sleeve Surgery Requires Resilience, Commitment, And Ongoing Support. Individuals May Face Various Physical, Emotional, And Lifestyle Challenges During The Recovery Process. Here Are Strategies To Help Overcome Common Challenges:

1. Nutritional Challenges:

• **Challenge:** Adapting To A New Diet, Meeting Protein Goals, And Managing Portion Sizes Can Be Challenging.

Strategies:

• Work Closely With A Registered Dietitian For Personalized Guidance And Support.

• Experiment With Nutrient-Dense Foods To Ensure Optimal Nutrition.

• Use Meal Planning And Portion Control Techniques.

• Incorporate A Variety Of Textures And Flavors To Make Meals More Enjoyable.

2. Hydration Difficulties:

• **Challenge:** Ensuring Adequate Hydration Can Be Challenging, Leading To Potential Issues Like Dehydration.

Strategies:

• Carry A Water Bottle and Sip Regularly Throughout the Day.

• Infuse Water With Natural Flavors Like Citrus Or Herbs For Variety.

• Monitor Urine Color As A Simple Indicator Of Hydration Status.

• Limit Caffeine And Sugary Beverage Intake.

3. Emotional And Psychological Challenges:

• **Challenge:** Dealing With Emotional Aspects Such As Body Image Changes, Adjusting To A New Lifestyle, And Potential Emotional Eating.

Strategies:

• Seek Support From Mental Health Professionals, Support Groups, Or Friends And Family.

• Practice Self-Compassion and Focus on Non-Scale Victories.

• Develop Healthy Coping Mechanisms For Stress Or Emotional Challenges.

• Engage In Activities That Bring Joy And Fulfillment.

4. Physical Activity Hurdles:

• **Challenge:** Gradually Reintroducing And Maintaining Physical Activity Can Be Challenging Due To Physical Limitations.

Strategies:

• Start With Low-Impact Activities Such As Walking And Gradually Increase Intensity.

• Consult With Healthcare Professionals For Tailored Exercise Recommendations.

• Find Enjoyable Activities To Make Exercise A Positive Part Of Your Routine.

• Incorporate Strength Training To Preserve And Build Muscle Mass.

5. Social and Lifestyle Adjustments:

• **Challenge:** Navigating Social Situations, Dining Out, And Managing Lifestyle Changes.

Strategies:

- Communicate Openly With Friends And Family About Your Dietary Needs.

- Choose Restaurants With Healthier Options And Smaller Portion Sizes.

- Participate In Social Activities That Don't Revolve Solely Around Food.

- Develop Strategies For Handling Peer Pressure Related To Eating.

6.   Plateaus   and   Weight Fluctuations:

- **Challenge:** Experiencing Weight Plateaus Or Fluctuations Can Be Discouraging.

Strategies:

- Focus On Non-Scale Victories, Such As Improved Energy Levels Or Clothing Fit.

- Reevaluate Dietary And Exercise Habits With The Guidance Of Healthcare Professionals.

- Understand That Weight Loss May Not Be Linear, And Plateaus Are A Normal Part Of The Process.

- Celebrate Achievements And Milestones Along The Way.

7. Surgical Complications:

- **Challenge:** Dealing With Potential Surgical Complications Or Unexpected Issues.

Strategies:

• Report Any Unusual Symptoms or Concerns Promptly To Healthcare Professionals.

• Attend Regular Follow-Up Appointments To Monitor Progress And Address Issues.

• Be Proactive In Seeking Medical Attention For Any Signs Of Complications.

8. Long-Term Commitment:

• **Challenge:** Maintaining Long-Term Commitment To Lifestyle Changes And Healthy Habits.

Strategies:

• Set Realistic And Achievable Goals For The Short And Long Term.

• Build A Support System With Healthcare Professionals, Friends, And Family.

• Revisit And Adjust Goals As Needed To Stay Motivated.

• Focus On The Overall Improvement In Health And Well-Being.

9. Self-Care and Mindfulness:

• **Challenge:** Balancing Self-Care And Mindfulness To Support Overall Well-Being.

Strategies:

• Prioritize Self-Care Activities, Including Adequate Sleep, Relaxation, And Stress Management.

• Practice Mindfulness Techniques Such As Meditation Or Deep Breathing.

• Identify And Address Emotional Triggers That May Lead To Unhealthy Habits.

10. Regular Follow-Up and Support:

• **Challenge:** Maintaining Regular Follow-Up Appointments And Seeking Ongoing Support.

Strategies:

• Attend Scheduled Check-Ups With Healthcare Professionals.

• Engage In Support Groups Or Counseling For Continued Guidance.

• Celebrate Achievements And Share Challenges With Your Support Network.

• Stay Proactive In Seeking Assistance When Needed.

Overcoming Challenges After Gastric Sleeve Surgery Is A Gradual Process That Requires Patience, Persistence, And A Holistic Approach To Health. Seeking Professional Guidance, Building A Strong Support System, And Prioritizing Self-Care Contribute To A Successful And Sustainable Postoperative Journey.

Incorporating Exercise Into Your Routine

Incorporating Exercise Into Your Routine After Gastric Sleeve Surgery Is An Essential Aspect Of Maintaining Overall Health, Supporting Weight Management, And Preserving Muscle Mass. However, It's Crucial To Approach Exercise Gradually And In Consultation With Your Healthcare Team To Ensure Safety And Effectiveness. Here Are Guidelines For Incorporating Exercise Into Your Postoperative Routine:

1.   Consult   With   Healthcare Professionals:

• **Clearance:** Obtain Clearance From Your Surgeon Or Healthcare Provider Before Starting Any Exercise Program.

• **Individualized Plan:** Work With A Physical Therapist Or Fitness Professional To Create An Individualized Exercise Plan Based On Your Health Status, Fitness Level, And Any Surgical Restrictions.

2. Start Slowly:

• **Gradual Progression:** Begin With Low-Intensity Exercises And Gradually Increase The Intensity And Duration As Your Fitness Level Improves.

• Listen To Your Body: Pay Attention To How Your Body Responds To Exercise. If You Experience Pain, Discomfort, Or Unusual Symptoms, Modify Or Stop The Activity And Consult With Your Healthcare Team.

3. Types of Exercise:

• Aerobic Exercise:

• Start With Low-Impact Activities Like Walking, Swimming, Or Stationary Cycling.

• Gradually Increase The Intensity And Duration Of Aerobic Exercises.

- **Strength Training:**

- Incorporate Resistance Training Using Light Weights Or Resistance Bands.

- Focus On All Major Muscle Groups To Preserve And Build Lean Muscle Mass.

- **Flexibility and Stretching:**

- Include Stretching Exercises To Improve Flexibility And Prevent Stiffness.

- Perform Dynamic Stretches Before Exercise And Static Stretches Afterward.

4. Frequency and Duration:

- **Consistency Is Key:** Aim For At Least 150 Minutes Of Moderate-Intensity Aerobic Exercise Per Week, Spread Over Most Days.

- **Strength Training:** Include Strength Training Exercises At Least Two Days A Week.

5. Postoperative Considerations:

- **Avoid High-Impact Activities:** Limit Activities That May Put Excess Stress On The Joints, Especially In The Early Stages Of Recovery.

- **Mindful Movements:** Engage In Mindful Movements And Exercises That Promote Body Awareness.

6. Work On Core Strength:

• **Gentle Core Exercises:** Incorporate Gentle Core-Strengthening Exercises To Support Your Abdominal Muscles.

• **Pilates Or Yoga:** Consider Pilates Or Yoga For Core Strength, Flexibility, And Relaxation.

7. Stay Hydrated:

• **Fluid Intake: Stay** Well-Hydrated Before, During, And After Exercise, Especially Considering The Potential Changes In Fluid Balance Post-Surgery.

8. Modify Based On Tolerance:

• **Individual Tolerance:** Modify Exercises Based On Your Individual

Tolerance And Any Feedback From Your Healthcare Team.

• **Progress Gradually:** As You Become More Comfortable With Exercise, Gradually Progress To More Challenging Activities.

9. Make It Enjoyable:

• **Choose Activities You Enjoy:** Select Activities That You Find Enjoyable To Enhance Adherence To Your Exercise Routine.

• **Variety:** Keep Your Routine Varied To Prevent Boredom And Target Different Muscle Groups.

10. Social Support:

• Exercise Partners: Consider Exercising With A Friend Or Joining A Group To Provide Motivation And Support.

• **Accountability:** Having Someone To Share Your Fitness Journey With Can Increase Accountability.

11. Regular Check-Ups:

• Follow-Up Appointments: Attend Regular Check-Ups With Your Healthcare Team To Monitor Your Progress And Make Any Necessary Adjustments To Your Exercise Routine.

12. Celebrate Progress:

• Acknowledge Achievements: Celebrate Your Achievements, Whether It's Reaching A Specific Milestone Or Consistently Sticking To Your Exercise Routine.

• Non-Scale Victories: Focus On Non-Scale Victories Such As Increased Energy Levels, Improved Mood, And Enhanced Mobility.

Remember That The Key To Successful And Sustainable Exercise After Gastric Sleeve Surgery Is To Start Slowly, Progress Gradually, And Prioritize Consistency. Always Consult With Your Healthcare Team Before Initiating Any Exercise Program, And

Make Adjustments Based On Your Individual Needs And Tolerance. Exercise Should Enhance Your Overall Well-Being And Contribute To A Healthy And Active Lifestyle.

Conclusion

After Gastric Sleeve Surgery, The Trip Is A Transforming And Continuous Process That Requires Adjusting To New Lifestyle Patterns, Accepting Change, And Focusing On Overall Well-Being. Success Requires A Holistic Approach To Nutrition, Consistent Exercise, Emotional Well-Being, And Lifestyle Changes. Collaborating Closely With Healthcare Professionals Such As Nutritionists, Surgeons, And Mental Health Experts Is Essential To Guarantee A Customized And Secure Postoperative Journey.

Success Recipes Stress The Significance Of Incremental Advancement, Personalized Attention,

And A Happy Attitude. Portion Control, Attentive Eating, And Staying Hydrated Are Crucial For Aiding The Recuperation Process. Engaging In Various Forms Of Exercise, Such As Aerobic Activities, Weight Training, And Flexibility Exercises, Benefits Both Physical Health And Emotional Well-Being.

Recognizing Accomplishments, Appreciating Successes Beyond Weight Loss, And Building A Strong Support System Of Friends And Family Are Crucial Aspects Of A Successful Recovery After Surgery. Long-Term Success And Overall Well-Being Are Enhanced By Flexibility, Adaptability,

And A Dedication To Constant Learning.

It Is Crucial For Individuals To Attend Regular Follow-Up Consultations With Healthcare Specialists, Evaluate Nutrient Levels, And Make Any Alterations To Their Plan In Order To Achieve Sustained Success After Surgery. Engaging In Self-Care Activities Such As Sufficient Sleep, Relaxation, And Consistent Self-Assessment Improves One's Overall Quality Of Life.

Each Person's Journey Is Distinct, And There Is No Universal Solution. The Period Following Gastric Sleeve Surgery Presents A Chance For Personal Development, Self-

Exploration, And The Fostering Of A Better And More Satisfying Lifestyle. By Combining The Correct Components And Adopting A Holistic Approach To Health, People Can Reach Their Weight And Health Objectives And Flourish After Surgery.

THE END